pink tips.
breast cancer advice from someone who's been there.

"This poignant book will help millions the way her documentary, 'The Breast Cancer Diaries,' has." New York Times Bestselling Author Lee Woodruff.

Ann Murray Paige

pink tips.

breast cancer advice from someone who's been there.

by Ann Murray Paige

"This poignant book will help millions the way her documentary, 'The Breast Cancer Diaries,' has." New York Times Bestselling Author Lee Woodruff.

A portion of the sale of this book goes to the non-profit
Project Pink,
help and hope for young women
with breast cancer.
www.projectpinkdiary.com

Also by Ann Murray Paige:

Words To Live By
More Words to Live By (Fall, 2011)
The Face of Breast-less America; A Memoir (Spring, 2012)
"The Breast Cancer Diaries" DVD (2005)

For purchase and advanced sales, go to
www.annmurraypaige.com

Author's Note

When I decided to put this book together people thought it should be for a certain audience. They suggested it be either for the cancer patients themselves or for all the people trying to support the cancer patient. I tried to follow that advice but found it difficult because so much of what I learned during my breast cancer journey had a lot to do with what I needed and got from my supportive family and friends. It became impossible for me to try to separate the two worlds. So this book is for all of us: those diagnosed with breast cancer (or any cancer for that matter) and all those who love us.

I hope it gives you hope and help on your breast cancer journey.

-Ann Murray Paige
  May 2011

FOR SANDY

FORWARD

In the spring of 2004 I was diagnosed with Stage 2 breast cancer. At age 38 with a husband, 2 children and a television journalism career in the balance, I was devastated by this surprise diagnosis.

One of the first things people did was buy me books. I received books about breast cancer, healing breast cancer, getting breast cancer and living past breast cancer. But I was in no shape to sit down and read a thick book. I needed quick answers. I wanted Cancer Cliff Notes.

9 months later, after surgery, chemotherapy and radiation, I realized I'd learned more about breast cancer and getting through it than I ever wanted to know. I sat down and penned what I'd learned and what the things were that got me through my ordeal. I also co-founded Project Pink, a non-profit that brings help and hope to young women with breast cancer and all who love them. I began posting my top breast cancer survival tips at www.projectpinkdiary.com.

In the following weeks and months so many people--the newly diagnosed, the friends of the diagnosed, and survivors themselves--asked for the rest of my tips or how they could "buy the book" that I decided to write "the book"--and this is it.

My children are growing, my husband and I are happily married and I am grateful for every day I am here in this world. And still almost daily I receive emails and phone calls from people I know whose friend, sister, mother, wife, aunt, cousin, niece or neighbor has just been diagnosed with breast cancer--or worse, they have it themselves . They ask me, *what now?*

This book is my answer. It's a fast look at the worst year of my life; it's hard won insight that I hope is helpful to anyone embroiled in this same ugly fight.

And fight we must.

-Ann Murray Paige

1. **go ahead and panic**.

I am giving everyone permission to flip out.
Breast cancer is scary, no matter what.
People want to believe "it's going to be okay"
and it probably will be, but in the moments
after you get the news, it's terrifying. It's
okay to be scared.

"It's not the size of the dog in the fight. It's the size of
the fight in the dog."
-Dwight D. Eisenhower (1890-1969) American
President.

2. **stop panicking**.

Now that you've freaked out, stop. Cancer will be what it will be, and nobody knows what that is right now. You have to find your calm, find out what's in store from your doctor and proceed with courage, grace and hope.

"When you're going through Hell, keep going."
-*Winston Churchill (1874-1965)*
British Prime Minister.

3. **just show up**.

A breast cancer diagnosis can take two tones: either 'this is impossible' or 'I've no time for this'. But you can do this. And you must do this because the world needs you in it. If you have the cancer, you must beat it. If you are the friend, you can help. You don't have to have all the answers or figure it all out. You just have to show up for the fight.

"Success is not in getting a winning hand, but in playing a bad hand well."
-*Robert Louis Stevenson (1850-1894)*
  Scottish author and poet.

4. **all cancers are not made equal**.

You will hear about new drugs to battle breast cancer but realize these latest drugs often target a specific population of patients. Cancers are different depending on your age, disease stage and grade, and your family history. Ask the doctor what you're dealing with so you don't get all confused about what's next.

"I can be changed by what happens to me, but I refuse to be reduced by it."
-Maya Angelou (b. 1928)
 American author and poet.

5. **do ask, do tell**.

When you're up against breast cancer, laundry seems ridiculous. And who cares how many dishes are in the sink when life has become so unpredictable? If you need help, ask for it. And if you can give help, give it.

"Remember my sentimental friend, that a heart is not judged by how much you love, but by how much you are loved by others.
-*The Wizard of Oz to the Tin Man*
  (MGM's "The Wizard of Oz".)

6. **just say no**.

A cancer diagnosis makes you very truthful. Suddenly saying how you truly feel isn't verboten and is even imperative. If you can't take any more visits from people just say so. And if you can't give any more visits that's okay too--cancer is intense. Take a break.

"You may have to fight a battle more than once to win."
-*Margaret Thatcher (b. 1925)*
British Prime Minister.

7. **get it off your chest**.

I mean the conversation you have to have with yourself and your partner about a possible mastectomy. Ask your doctor what the medical chances are of recurrence in every option; lumpectomy, mastectomy and prophylactic mastectomy. And be sure you'd feel good about the decision should your cancer return. I chose a prophylactic bilateral mastectomy with no reconstruction to keep invasions to my body to a minimum. This was not an easy decision but to quote my husband, "I just want you healthy. We'll figure out the rest."

"Taking joy in living is a woman's best cosmetic."
~Rosalind Russell (1907-1976)
 American actress.

8. **like the doctor**.

If you don't, find another one. This is not the time to worry about hurting somebody's feelings. Consult trusted people and do research on all options before making a medical choice. And if after meeting this person (or after several meetings) you find you don't like what's going on, find a new doctor. Comfort with your medical team is critical for healing.

"Sometimes courage does not roar. Sometimes it is the quiet voice at the end of the day saying I will try again tomorrow."
-*Maryanne Radmacher (b. ?)*
American writer.

9. **beware the internet**.

Yes, it's got lots of advice and tons of resources, but sometimes too much of a good thing is too much. Many times what's on the Internet is scary and isn't even relevant to you or your loved one's situation. Ask the doctor about what you've researched so you can separate what's a real concern from what's commonly know as TMI--too much information. (And try waiting until the morning of your appointment before you surf the Net so you don't spend days fearing the worst.)

"Only a fool tests the waters with both feet."
-African Proverb.

10. **write it down**.

The information in a doctor's session comes fast and hearing all this medical jargon can be overwhelming. Write questions down before you get to the doctor's waiting room so you don't forget. And if you're alone, record your doctor's sessions so you can remember what was said later on. Cancer news is frightening and the brain can turn off when it gets overwhelmed--press record/play to make it easier.

"You can do it. We can help."
-Home Depot
 American home improvement store.

11. **let it out**.

A social worker told me it's impossible to go over or under a cancer diagnosis; you have to go through it. She encouraged me to let out my fears so I could move through them to the next emotions. When I did I was happily surprised to discover better emotions waiting for me on the other side--like determination, bravery and courage.

"We must build dikes of courage to hold back the flood of fear."
-Martin Luther King Jr. (1929-1968)
African-American leader.

12. **forget yourself**.

Take an afternoon off from breast cancer. Sit in a bookstore (in the comedy aisle,) go to a movie, out to lunch, hang with pals and pretend you're somebody else without a care in the world. If only for an hour, check your disease at the door. This cancer stuff is intense and you deserve a day off.

"Breakdowns can create breakthroughs. Things fall apart so things can fall together."
-*Author Unknown*.

13. **be honest**.

So often when someone gets sick, the person who's ill feels weird about it and the friends around them do too. That's okay, and it's okay to admit it. Saying "this is awkward" to your friend, partner, or yourself is so much better than pretending nothing's wrong.

"They can because they think they can."
-*Virgil (70 BC-19 BC)*
 Roman poet.

14. **cover up**.

Chemotherapy and radiation are hard on a body. Wear hats and sunscreen to give your epidermis protection. If you lose your hair to chemotherapy know that a wig can be hot and itchy. There are many soft and stylish options for head wraps and do-rags in hospital gift stores, on the Internet or in regular department store scarf shelves. (Note: not all chemotherapy makes hair fall out. Ask your doctor so you'll know what's ahead.)

"The ideal man bears the accidents of life with dignity and grace, making the best of circumstances."
-*Aristotle (384 BC-322 BC)*
 Greek philosopher.

15. **go commando**.

I don't mean underwear, I'm talking about your head. Every now and then it's important to look a bald head in the face and appreciate all it symbolizes: the fight, the courage, the strength and the determination to succeed.

"Facing it, always facing it, that's the way to get through. Face it."
-Joseph Conrad (1857-1924)
 British novelist.

16. **rock on**.

Money may make the world go around, but music really drives the beat. There are times when the difficulty of the cancer experience makes most things too much to bear. But listening is always easy, and there's nothing like a favorite tune to calm the nerves and massage the soul.

"The proof of gold is fire."
-Benjamin Franklin (1706-1790)
American statesman, scientist and philosopher.

17. **move it**.

Getting out to exercise, if only for 5 minutes, is a mental and medical boost. Walking, biking, swimming, or gardening are ways to get up and out of the house. Local tracks are a good indoor option for motion and if all else fails there's always the mall.

"The world breaks everyone and afterward many are stronger at the broken places."
-*Ernest Hemingway (1898-1961)*
American writer.

18. **hold hands**.

This may sound goofy but the feeling of someone else's hand translates to comfort. In the middle of a world falling apart, the human touch can help hold a life together.

"I'm not afraid of storms, for I'm learning to sail my ship."
-Louisa May Alcott (1832-1888)
 American author.

19. **lose the (bad) news**.

Dealing with cancer is bad news all day long. Piling on information about wars, famines, tornadoes and floods makes the bad news you're already dealing with in your world suffocatingly worse. Take a break from the sad headlines until strength (or world peace and the rain forest) return.

"A wounded deer leaps the highest."
-*Emily Dickinson (1830-1866)*
 American poet.

20. **find a good book**.

You've already found this one-but there are others that can guide without overwhelming. I liked "*Just Get Me Through This: A Practical Guide to Coping With Breast Cancer*." It was my cancer resource because it was funny, quick and gave me tips on how to avoid chemotherapy side effects.

"If you want happiness for an hour -- take a nap. If you want happiness for a day -- go fishing. If you want happiness for a month -- get married. If you want happiness for a year -- inherit a fortune. If you want happiness for a lifetime -- help someone else." *-Chinese Proverb.*

21. "domino's delivers."

The last thing I wanted to do after a busy day of cancer was cook. I don't like to cook either so this really worked for me--but if you enjoy cooking you may find you need to take a break from it to concentrate on your health. Take out food was the new food group in my house, and I was thrilled when dinners showed up at the door through a "friend's food chain" organized by my pals.

"The problem with cookbooks is they don't come with cooks."
-Ann Murray Paige (b. 1965)
(American breast cancer activist.)

22. **break out the Chinet**.

Buy tons of paper plates and don't worry about doing dishes. This is not eco-friendly but there are bigger things on the horizon now.   When all this is over you'll go back to saving the earth. Right now you have to save your sanity.

"To the world you may be one person, but to one person you may be the world."
-Author Unknown.

23. **money matters**.

When I was sick my children were 1 and 4 and my husband and I needed childcare help. Our families donated to a nanny fund. When my friend got breast cancer her family pooled resources to pay her mortgage. Extra cash is helpful for potential babysitting needs, groceries, a cleaning lady, a mortgage payment, or other unexpected cancer bills.

"To know that even one life has breathed easier because you have lived; this is to have succeeded."
-Ralph Waldo Emerson (1803-1882)
American poet.

24. take the HOV lane.

The idea of a High Occupancy Vehicle lane on what I call the Cancer Highway is a must because it means we cancer fighters are not alone. Two by two (or three) is the way to go when heading to the doctor, to radiation, chemotherapy, or any other medical-based trip. Because support means strength.

"I may not be able to change the wind, but I can adjust my sails."
-Author Unknown.

25. **keep talking**.

Whether it's one day after chemotherapy treatments are over or three months from a yearly check-up, just keep talking to stay healthy. Breast cancer is a life-changing event, to be processed for years to come. You'll change, your partner will change, your friends, your kids--in ways that may be good and some ways that may not. Seek professional help if you find the road gets hard to walk comfortably.

"Courage is grace under pressure."
-Ernest Hemingway (1898-1961)
American writer.

26. **no falsies** (and I don't mean breasts).

Cancer is the fatal reminder that being phony is a waste of life. Included in that is the fact that some friends, while well-meaning, are a drag on your energy and spirit. You need to surround yourself with healthy, supportive relationships and if a "friend" doesn't fit that bill you need to let them go. A cancer patient may find they lose some friendships during this time and that's hard--but right now it's more about you than your friend.

"The ultimate measure of a man is not where he stands in moments of comfort and convenience, but where he stands at times of challenge and controversy."
-*Martin Luther King Jr. (1929-1968)*
 African-American leader.

27. **get falsies** (and I mean breasts).

I didn't get reconstructive surgery after my double mastectomy so I was offered pretend breasts. This was important to my grieving process even if I only wore them twice. And it was yet another bonding moment for me and my pals because you know who your friends are when they show up to help you choose your chest.

"A smooth sea never made a skillful mariner."
-*English proverb*.

28. **go short.**

I got a really short hair cut to prepare myself and my family for what I'd look like during chemotherapy (remember--not all chemotherapy causes hair loss.) It helped us all get a feel for the inevitable. I even had a few people say that they "loved my new do" (and all I kept thinking was "wait'll you see my next one.")

"Adversity is a fact of life. It can't be controlled. What we can control is how we react to it."
-Unknown Source.

29. take pictures.

Believe it or not, this time will go by and then life will return to a more typical routine-- whatever that definition becomes for you. Take photos to remind yourselves what real bravery, courage, friendship and strength look like.

"Whatever you do, you need courage."
-Ralph Waldo Emerson (1803-1882)
American poet, essayist and lecturer.

30. **break the rules**.

I don't mean the law--but have some fun. I got a washable tattoo and let my kids put purple sand in the kiddie pool. Doing fun, crazy things brings life right out in front of our eyes and helps us celebrate that we are here.

"Remember what is important to you."
-Chinese saying.

31. **celebrate your milestones**.

Whether you've made it through the first week of cancer confusion or your treatments are completely over, throw a party--even if you're the only one there. Cancer taught me to never miss a chance to have fun. Surround yourself with love--family, friends and a big fat cake filled with candles counting the time you've dealt with all this. Then take a big, healthy breath of life-sustaining air and blow those candles O-U-T.

"Life can only be understood backwards, but it must be lived forward."
-*Soren Kierkegaard (1813-1855)*
 Danish philosopher and writer.

32. **respect radiation**.

When chemotherapy is over--if you needed it, that is, many people don't-- it's a big relief. But radiation isn't easy. It doesn't hurt physically--though it is tiring--but it is intimidating to be under a huge machine behind a door marked DANGER. Go with your partner or a friend if you can for support--and share your feelings so you're not facing this part of the journey alone.

"One day your life will flash before your eyes. Make sure it's worth watching."
-Unknown Source.

33. **laugh a little**.

Not at cancer, of course, and not at this situation. It isn't funny. But decades later, Seinfeld on DVD is still funny--to me. Whatever it is that creates laughter during this time in your life, spend time with it. (My son Christopher was 4 when I was diagnosed and at preschool he decided his name had too many letters in it. When I picked him up that day his art work was signed CHRIST.)

"Laughter is the shortest distance between two people."
-*Victor Borge (1909-2000)*
 Danish humorist and musician.

34. **seek alternate routes**.

There are non-medical therapies that can help alleviate cancer treatment side effects and in some cases hasten the success of medical treatments. Acupuncture (which stopped my hot flashes,) massage, yoga, meditation and spa treatments are just a few. Talk to your doctor about them and see what makes sense for you.

"A gem cannot be polished without friction, nor a man perfected without trials."
-*Chinese Proverb*.

35. **get organized**.

Life gets confusing in a cancer diagnosis and dates blur together. Buy an organizer or hook up your hand-held calendar to your computer to help you prepare for what's next. I had a huge day planner duct-taped to my fridge so friends and family would know what was next if I was napping or unable to remember where I put my organizer (which happened a lot.)

"Always bear in mind that your own resolution to succeed is more important than any one thing."
-*Abraham Lincoln (1809 - 1865)*
 American president.

36. **splurge**.

Shop for clothes, take a family trip, get a pedicure, or buy that new grill you've been eyeing. You deserve it. My hallway Pottery Barn throw rug arrived after chemotherapy treatment number 5 and I was ridiculously excited about it. Sometimes it really is the little things during a trying time that make a big difference.

"Everything changes, nothing remains without change."
-Buddha (563 BC-483 BC)
 Founder of Buddhism.

37. **tell the kids**.

There are always kids--they may be your own or your nieces, nephews, neighbors' kids, or friends of your kids--who wonder what's happening and can be frightened if they don't understand. My children were 4 and 1 when I was diagnosed and I read them "Kemo Shark" to prepare them for my physical changes (available at kidscope.org). The Center for Grieving Children can be found online and has a help list of what to do and say to young people. And don't ever hesitate to get professional help.

"It is not the strongest of the species that survive, nor the most intelligent, but the one most responsive to change."
-*Charles Darwin (1809-1882)*
 English Naturalist.

38. **pamper the partner**.

Those who care about cancer patients need attention, too. They are going through hell feeling powerless to make a difference, and there's a strange reverse jealousy that comes with watching one person in the house get so much attention. When someone asked me what he could do for me, I told him to take my husband out and buy him a beer. The attention he got that night was like medicine for him ---the beer helped too.

"One who gains strength by overcoming obstacles possesses the only strength which can overcome adversity."
-*Albert Schweitzer (1875-1965)*
German theologian, philosopher, and physician.

39. **write on**.

Even if you jot down a sentence or two, writing is medicinal. It lets out stuff inside your head that even spoken words can't do. You don't have to be a poet, but you are living life at its most intense. Capture what you're feeling and you'll have it to help you look back and remember how brave you've been. And you'll have it to help you look forward and inspire you for what's next in your life.

"A stumble may prevent a fall."
-*English proverb.*

40. **question authority**.

I don't mean you should be disrespectful--
but get a second medical opinion because
treatments for cancer morph every
day. There are new drugs, new treatments
and new ways of dealing with old cancers.
Keep finding out what's out there, keep
asking questions and be confident in your
treatment. Remember that you are the boss
and you can fire, hire or switch your medical
team any time you want.

"Fortune favors the brave."
-Publius Terence (195/185 BC- 159 BC)
Roman playwright.

41. **if it stains, it's good for you**.

Eating right is good for everybody, but since you've got an up-close look at cancer, this is especially pertinent now. The nutritionist at the hospital ran down the list of good fruits and vegetables and must have seen the "how am I gonna remember all those?" look in my eyes. She stopped and said, "if it stains, it's good for you." Now that I can remember.

"Life is really simple, but we insist on making it complicated."
-*Confucius (551 BC-497 BC)*
 Chinese thinker and philosopher.

42. **let it go**.

By "it" I mean control. Of course you have to get up every day and plan your strategy. But understand that much of a cancer journey is out of your control and you just have to wing it. Nobody plans to have cancer. But you can plan to make it through.

"Our greatest glory is not in never falling but in rising every time we fall."
-*Confucius (551 BC-479 BC)*
 Chinese thinker and philosopher.

43. **see a therapist**.

When cancer gets to you, lean on professionals for help. Hospitals have social workers, family practice doctors have names and numbers, and often times cancer centers have free resources. This is big stuff and it's okay to get help--and get some for your family, too. You may have the cancer but everyone who loves you is going through it with you.

"Present fears are less than horrible imaginings."
-William Shakespeare (1564-1616)
English poet and playwright.

44. **let it ring**.

Every now and then unplug the phone, turn off the cell, don't go to the door and don't look at your email. Just breathe.

"The best way out is always through."

-Robert Frost (1874-1963)
 American poet.

45. **smell the roses.**

As the saying goes, "stop and smell the roses" in life, but who actually does that? During cancer, I made myself walk into a garden and see what I was missing. And I began to cry, not that I'd missed it all these years as much as the fact that I was grateful to still be here to smell the roses in the first place.

"A wise man is he who does not grieve for the thing which he has not, but rejoices for those which he has."
-Epictetus (50-120)
 Greek philosopher.

46. **"just do it"** (Nike was right).

What are those things you've said you'll do that you just haven't done yet? Sky dive? Run a marathon? Write a book? Cancer pushed me in ways I didn't like, but this one I did like. I have a certain amount of time here on earth and I need to start doing what I hoped I would with this lifetime. You do, too. Start now.

"When you're finished changing, you're finished."
-Benjamin Franklin (1706-1790)
American statesman, scientist and philosopher.

47. **GPS yourself**.

Meet yourself where you are in this journey. The cancer trip is an up and down road-- some days you're strong and ready, other days you're weak and want to give up. Find out where you are on any given day emotionally and go from there.

"Love sought is good, but given unsought is better."
-William Shakespeare (1564-1616)
British poet and playwright.

48. **it's not your fault.**

I have no idea why you got breast cancer and I don't know why I did either. I am very sure though that it's not because you're too nice, too hard working, wear too much blue or never liked your mother. Ignore those who try to tell you this (or worse). Keep your head high, your shoulders straight, believe in you and kick this breast cancer's butt. Keep your eyes open and watch your health horizons. It's a beautiful view out there and it's waiting just for you.

"When you come to the end of all that you know you must believe in one of two things: you will either find legs to stand on or you will be given wings to fly."
-*Author Unknown.*

49. **have faith.**

Whether you're Christian, Buddhist, Jewish, Muslim, Agnostic or Atheist, have faith. This is one of those times when a bad thing has happened to a good person, and it's hard to live through without reaching to make some kind of sense of it. I do not believe I got my cancer for a reason but I do believe I found many important and life-changing things from it. That in and of itself gave me faith. Even if it's faith in yourself, have some. You can do this. God, Mohammed, Jesus, Allah, or the person looking back at you in the mirror can and will help get you through.

"Better to light one small candle than to curse the darkness."
-Chinese proverb.

50. **don't go it alone.**

You may want to shut out the world and just deal with this on your own. Don't. This is big and you are one person. Let yourself get help. The American Cancer Society is a good place to start. Local cancer centers and hospitals have a regional finger on the pulse of what's nearby to support you and your loved ones during this weird time. And there are plenty of groups on the Internet with emotional, domestic, physical, spiritual and medical information--all you have to do is search.

You are not alone--there are many of us out there who are in your same boat. Grab a life jacket and sail on. You can do this.

"Bad things happen. Good things endure."
-Ann Murray Paige.

QUOTATION REFERENCES:

1. WWW.QUOTATIONSPAGE.COM (http://
WWW.QUOTATIONSPAGE.COM)

2. WWW.INSPIRATIONAL-QUOTES.INFO/
SUCCESS-QUOTES.

3. HTML (http://WWW.INSPIRATIONAL-
QUOTES.INFO/SUCCESS-QUOTES.HTML)

4. http://blog.gaiam.com/quotes/authors/
henry-david-thoreau/51809

5. http://www.inspirationpeak.com/
kindness.html

Nike, Chinet, Home Depot, Pottery Barn and Domino's Pizza are trademarks and get my never ending gratitude for inadvertently helping me through the worst year of my life.

pink tips. breast cancer advice from someone who's been there.
by ann murray paige

Special thanks to Mary Yin Liu for editing this book.

Ann Murray Paige is an award-winning television journalist, writer, blogger and co-founder of the 501 (c)3 non-profit **Project Pink** (www.projectpinkdiary.com.) She travels around the world to raise awareness of the issue of young women and breast cancer. Her film, '*The Breast Cancer Diaries',* has won several awards and shows in countries including Israel, Sweden, Canada, the US and all of Latin America, where it airs as "*Diario De Mi Cancer.*" She is an expert blogger at Discovery Health, where her blog, "*Beyond The Breast Cancer Diaries*" has been translated into two languages. '*Ann's Diary,*' her blog at **Project Pink**, was named a Top Cancer Blog of 2010. In April, 2011, Ann was featured in Seth Godin's book project "*Tales of the Revolution: True Stories of People Who Are Poking the Box and Making a Difference.*" In her television career Ann was nominated for a regional Emmy for Outstanding Host and won a Maine Association of Broadcasters award for her non-stop coverage and bilingual skills uncovering the plight of local migrant workers. She divides her time between Maine and California, where she sits on several film festival advisory boards.